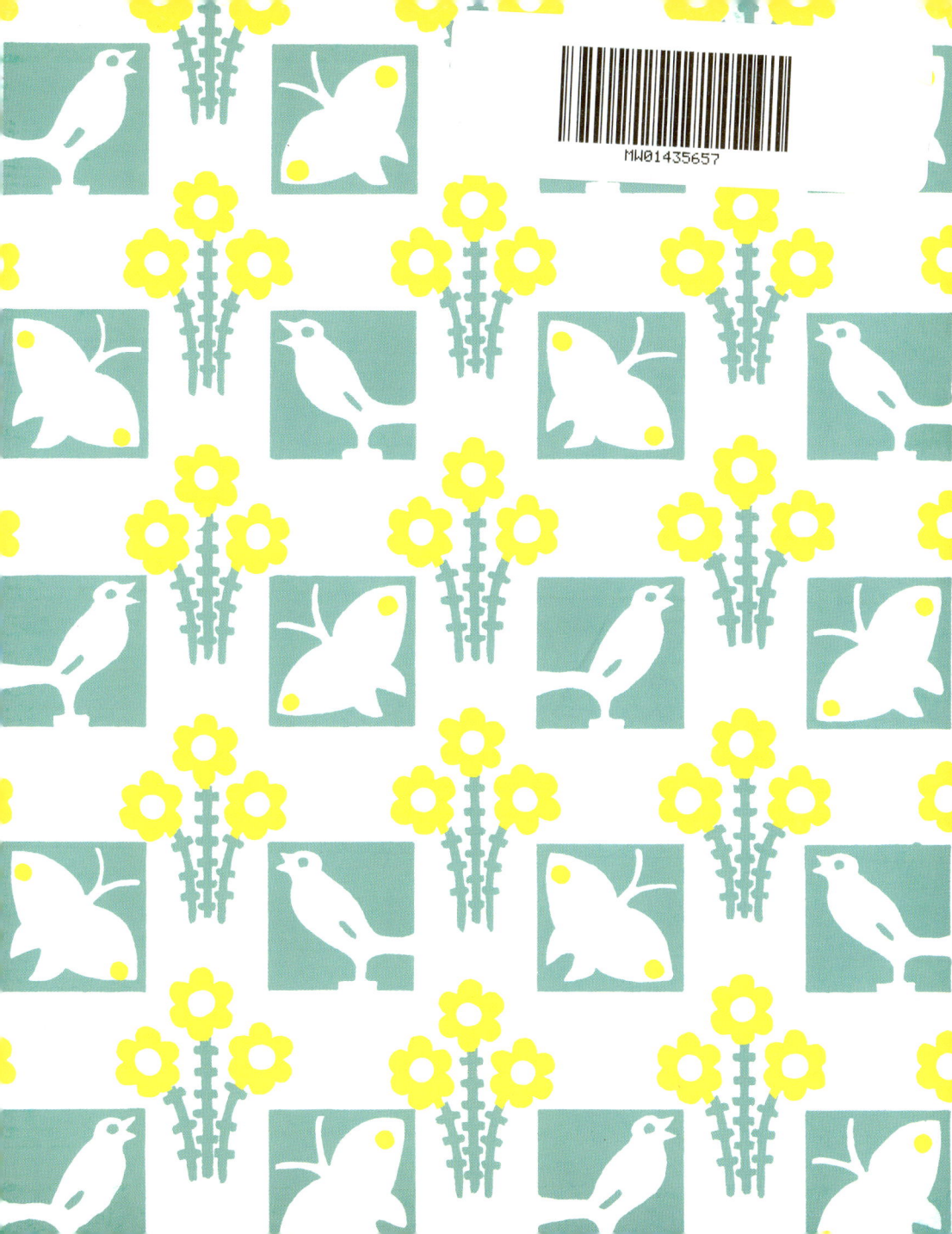

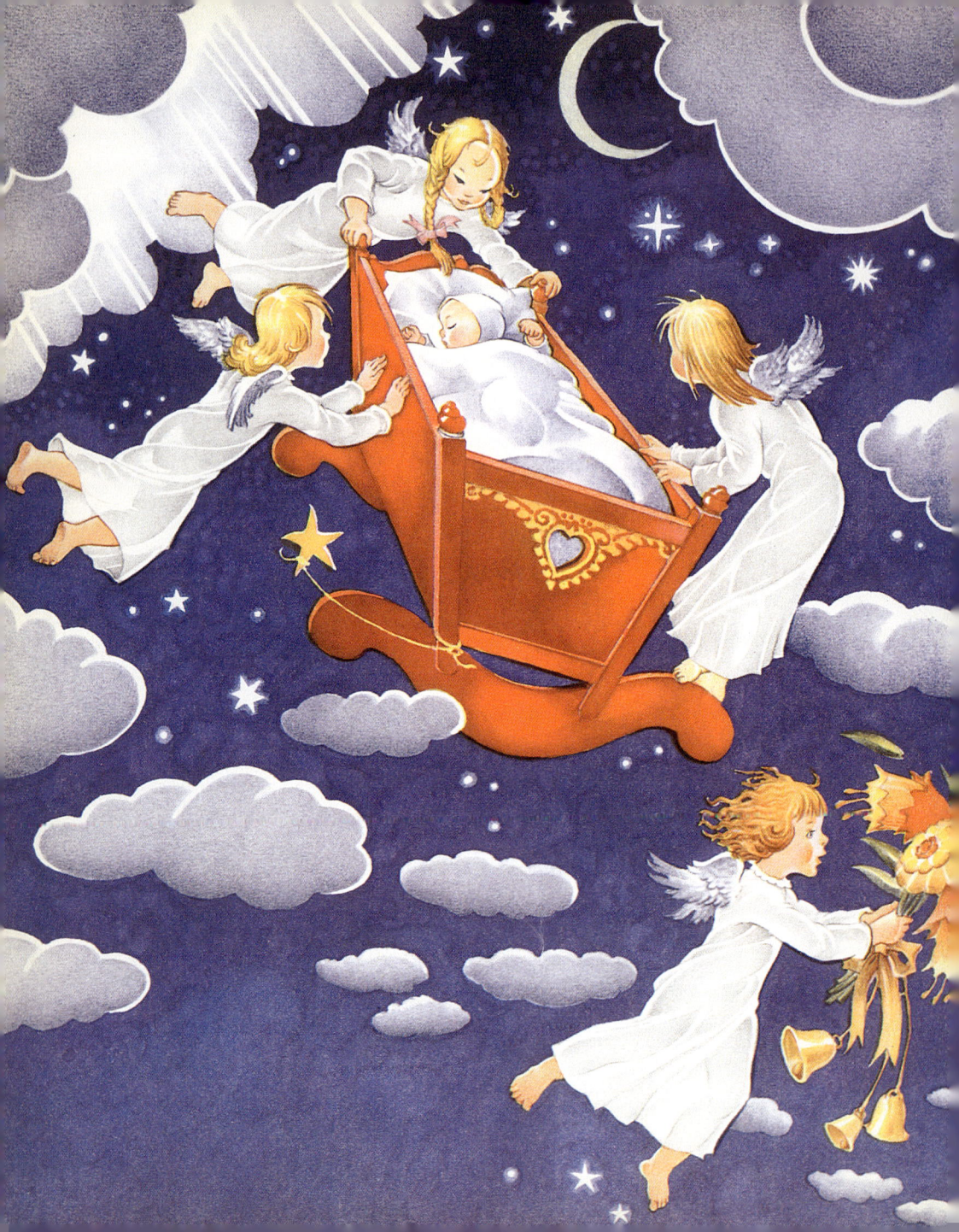

Welcome Baby

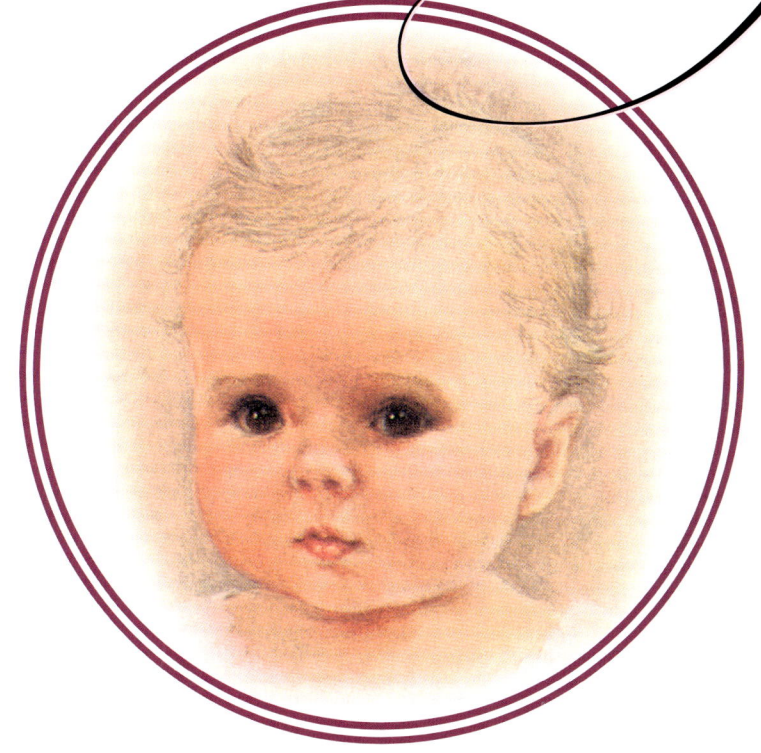

BY WELLERAN POLTARNEES

LAUGHING ELEPHANT

Baby Mia,

You are surrounded by so much love and kindness. We are very blessed to have you in our family. A wonderful, joyous life is ahead of you.

xoxo
Gigi
8/28/15

COPYRIGHT © 2004   BLUE LANTERN STUDIO

ISBN 1-59583-000-6

FIRST PRINTING   PRINTED IN CHINA THROUGH COLORCRAFT LTD., HONG KONG   ALL RIGHTS RESERVED

LAUGHING ELEPHANT BOOKS

3645 INTERLAKE AVENUE NORTH   SEATTLE   WASHINGTON   98103

WWW.LAUGHINGELEPHANT.COM

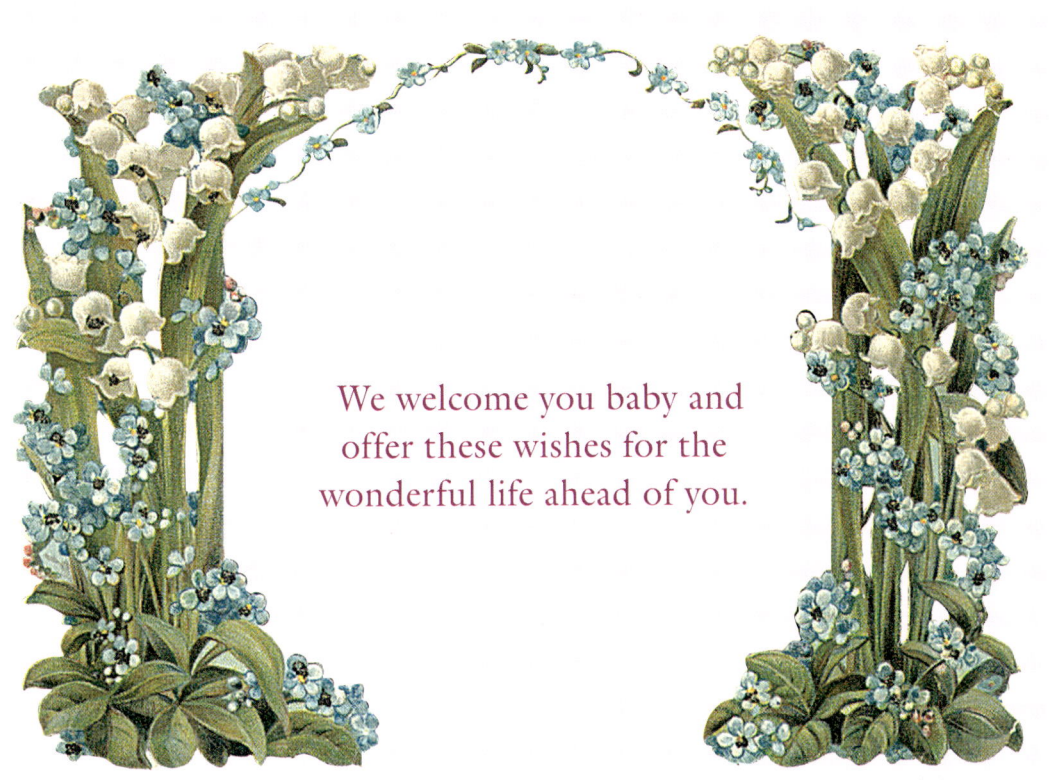

We welcome you baby and offer these wishes for the wonderful life ahead of you.

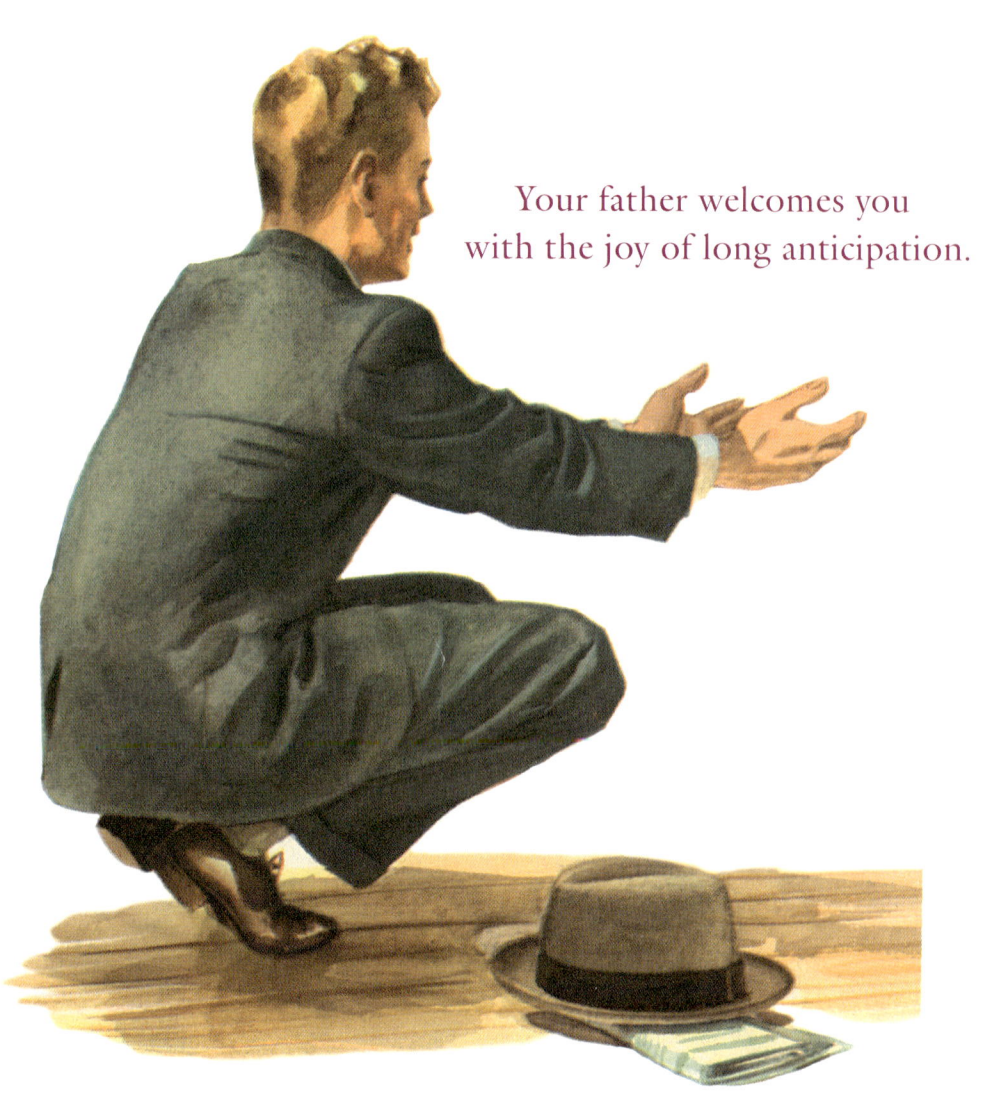

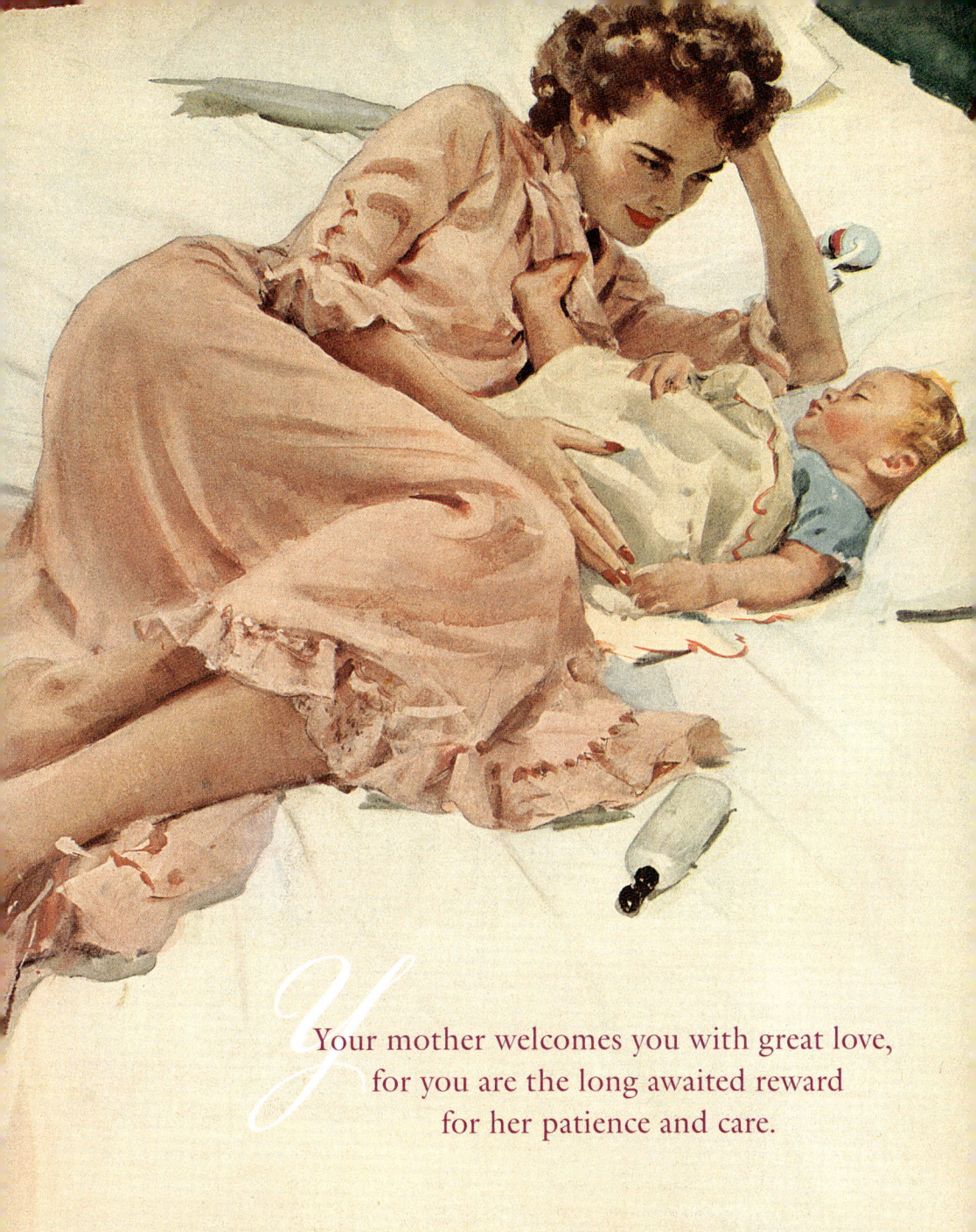

Your mother welcomes you with great love, for you are the long awaited reward for her patience and care.

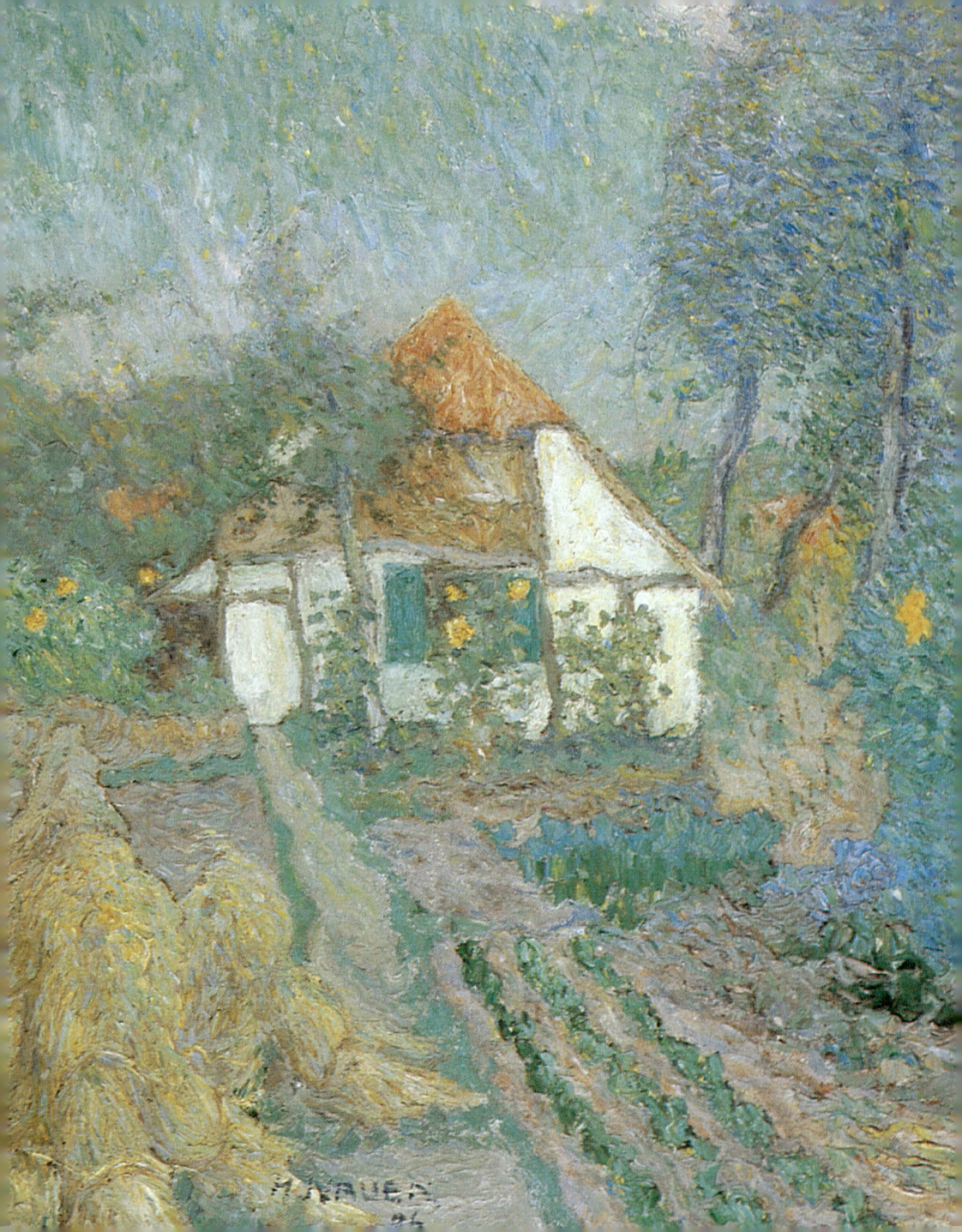

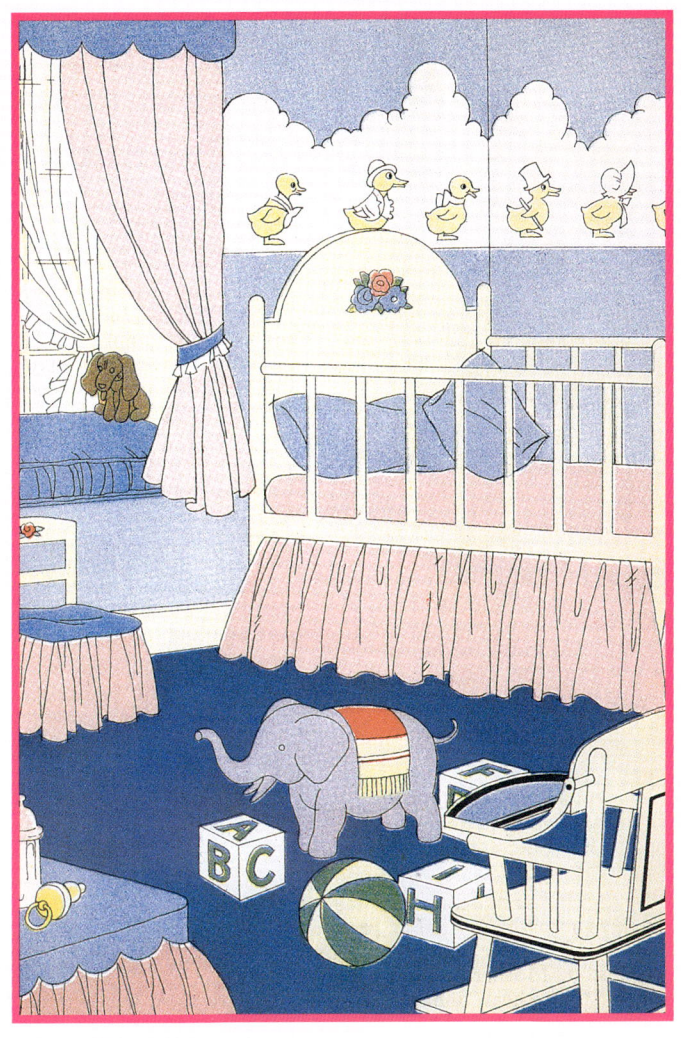

Your home will be a place of peace and caring nurture,

And your bed a small world of comfort and delight.

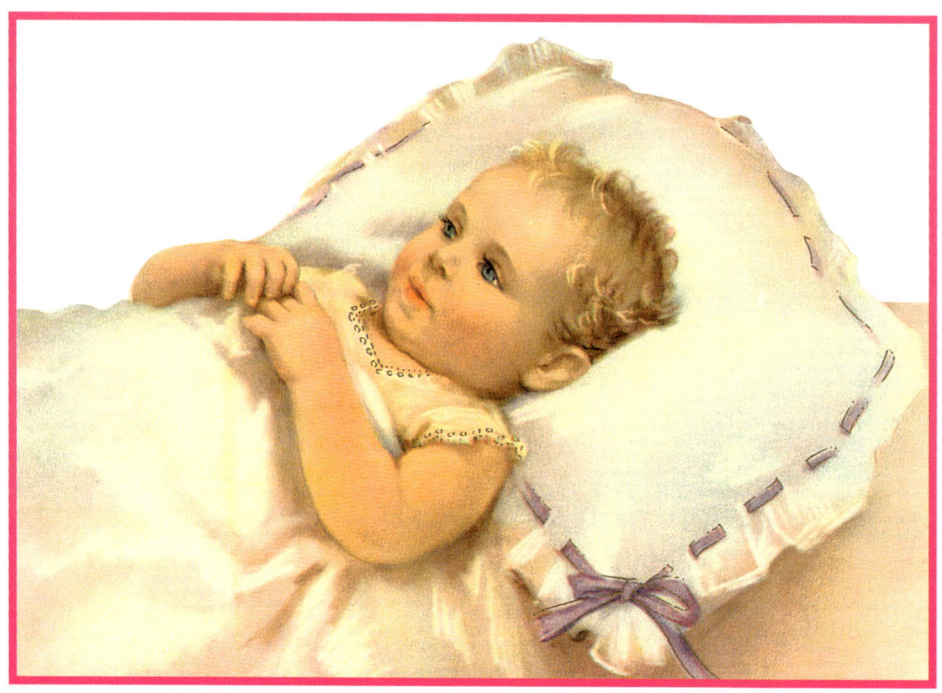

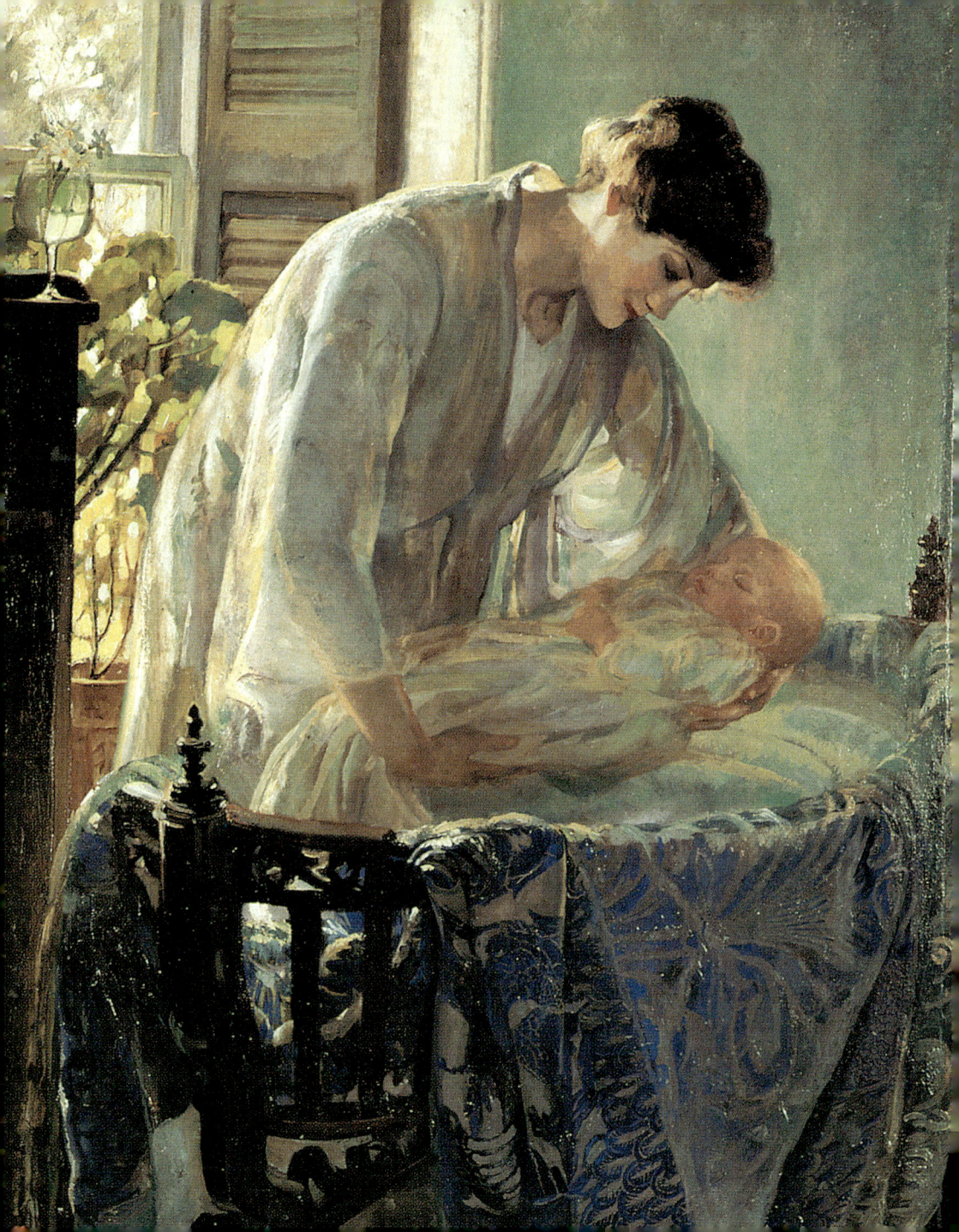

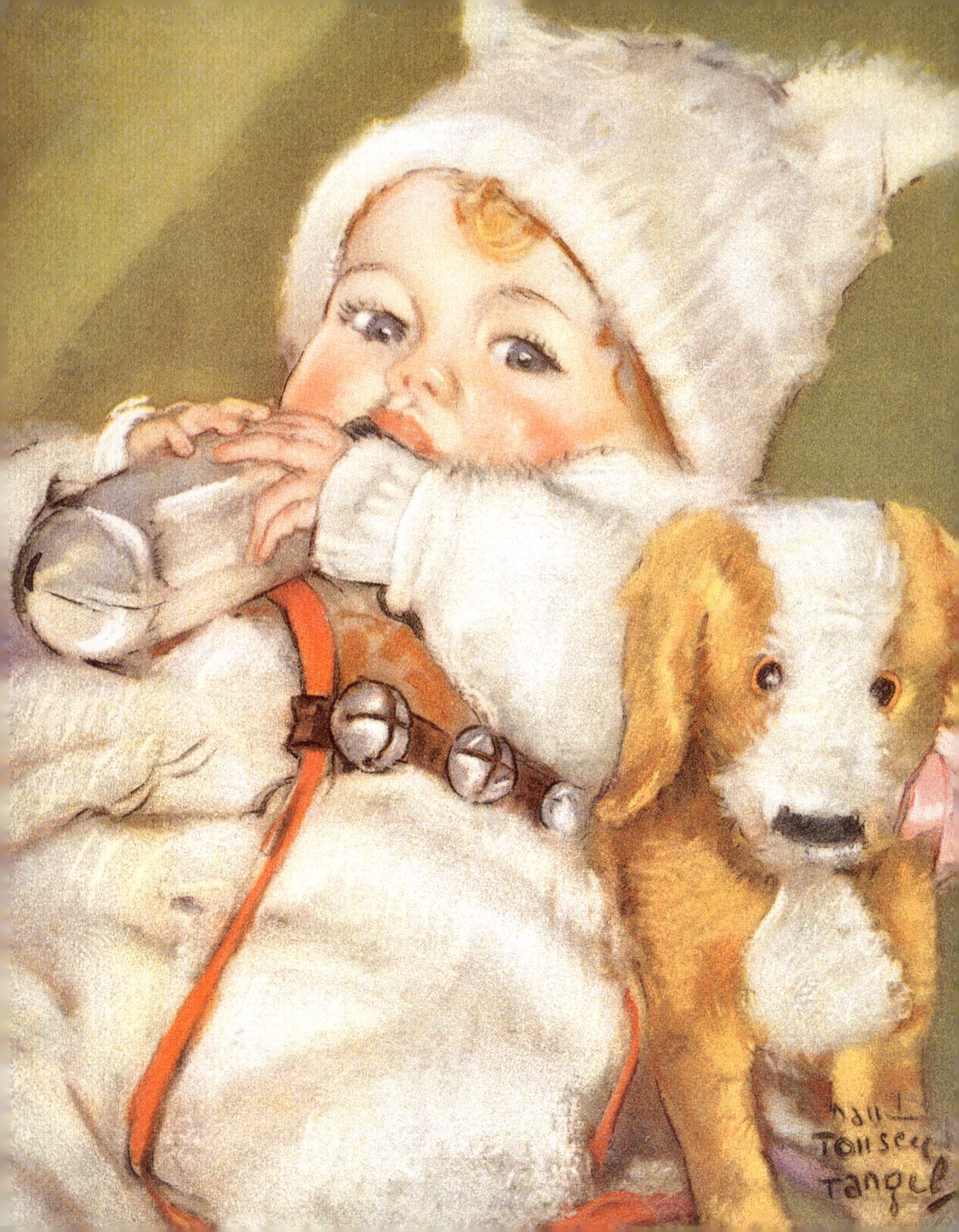

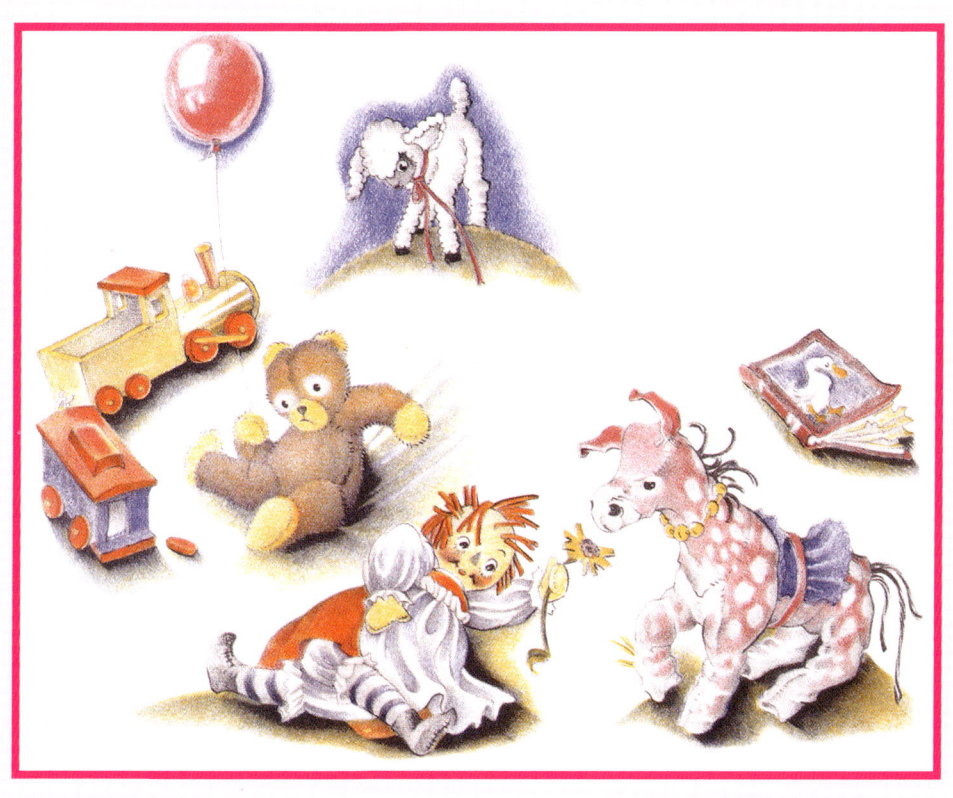

You will have uncountable good times,

And many friends to share them,

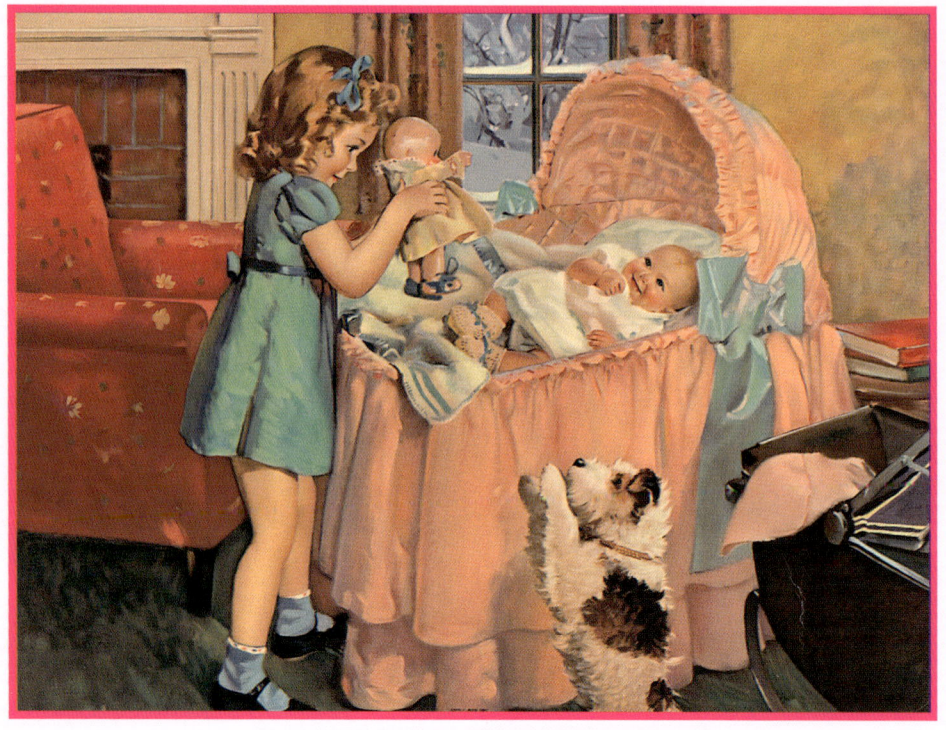

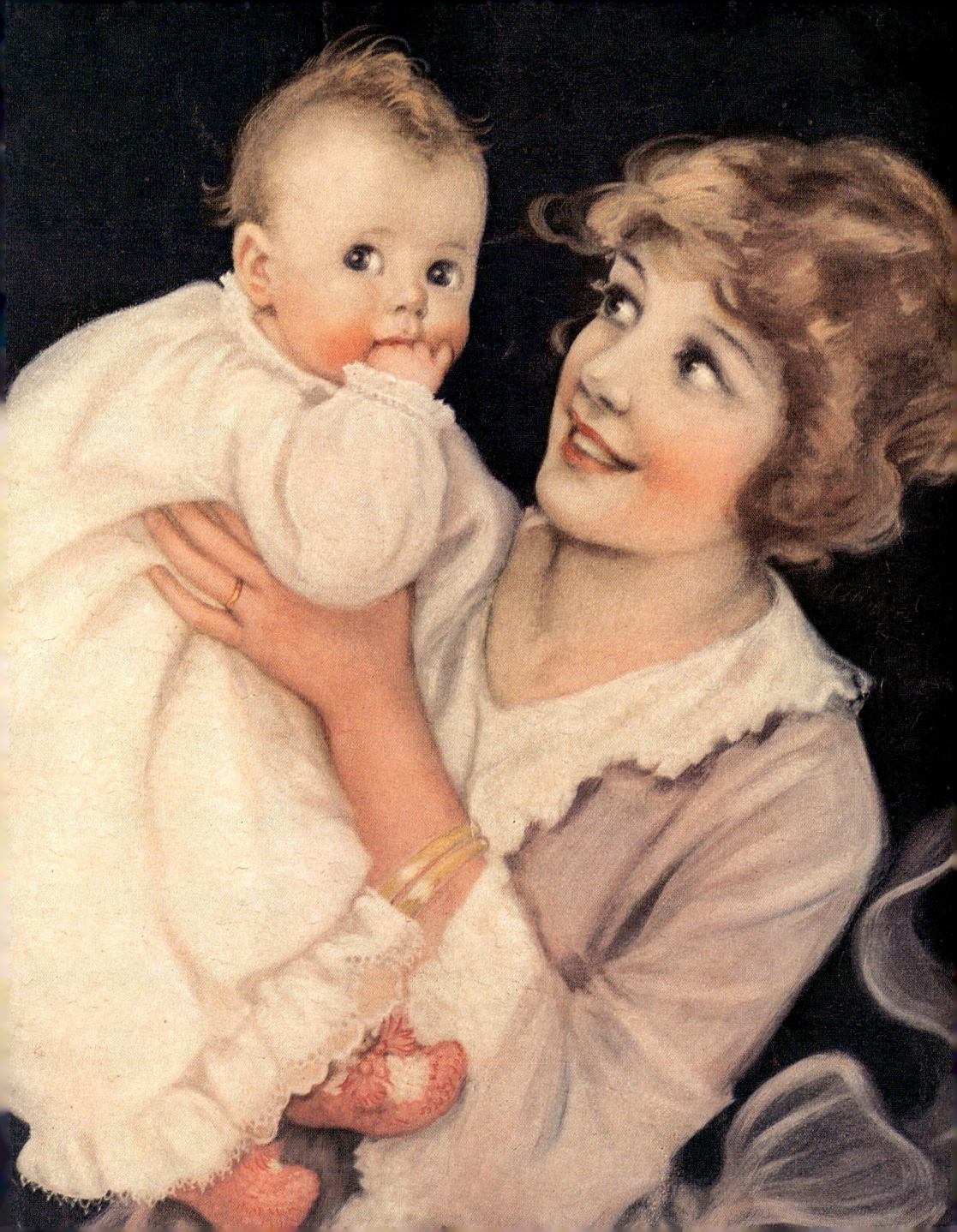

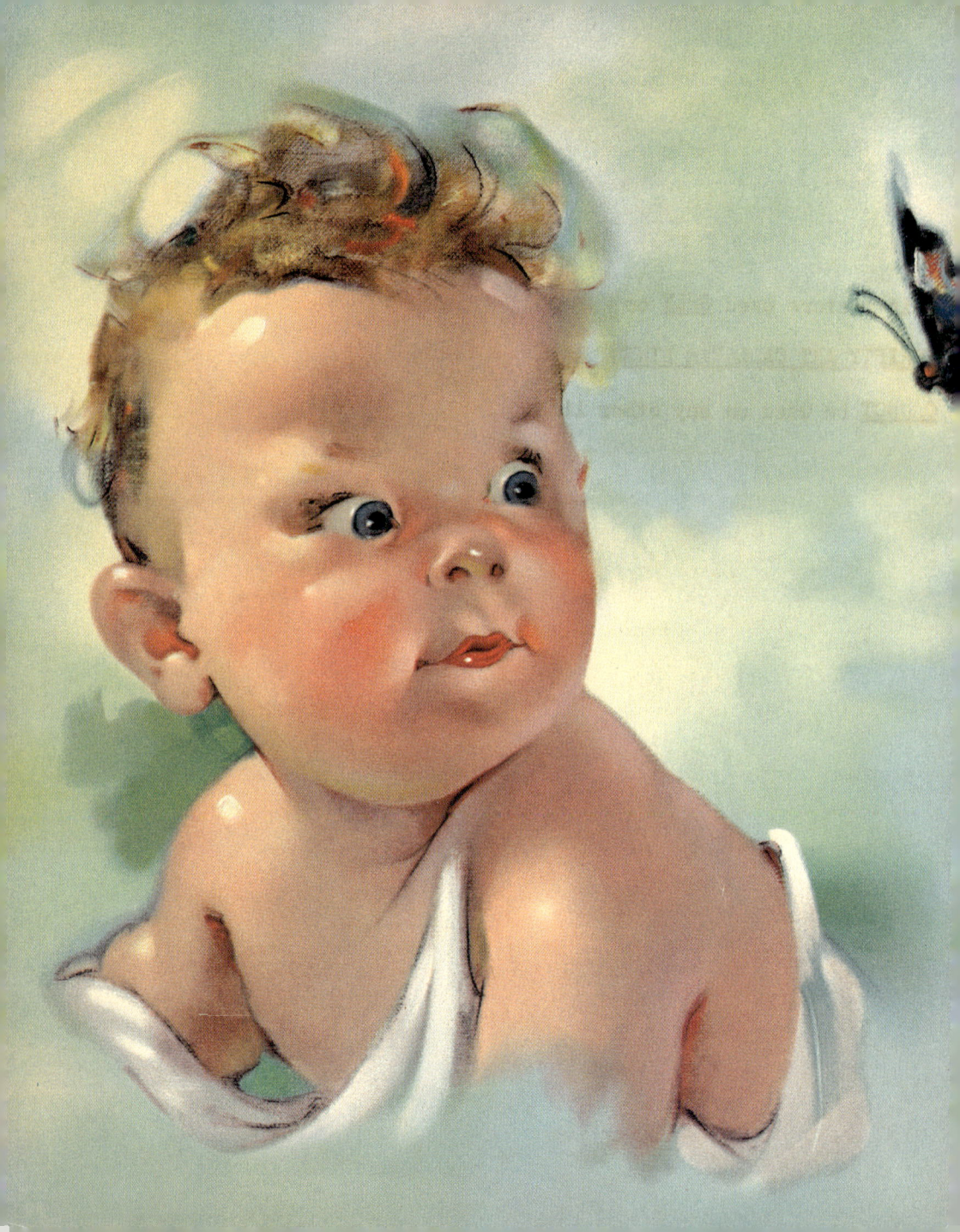

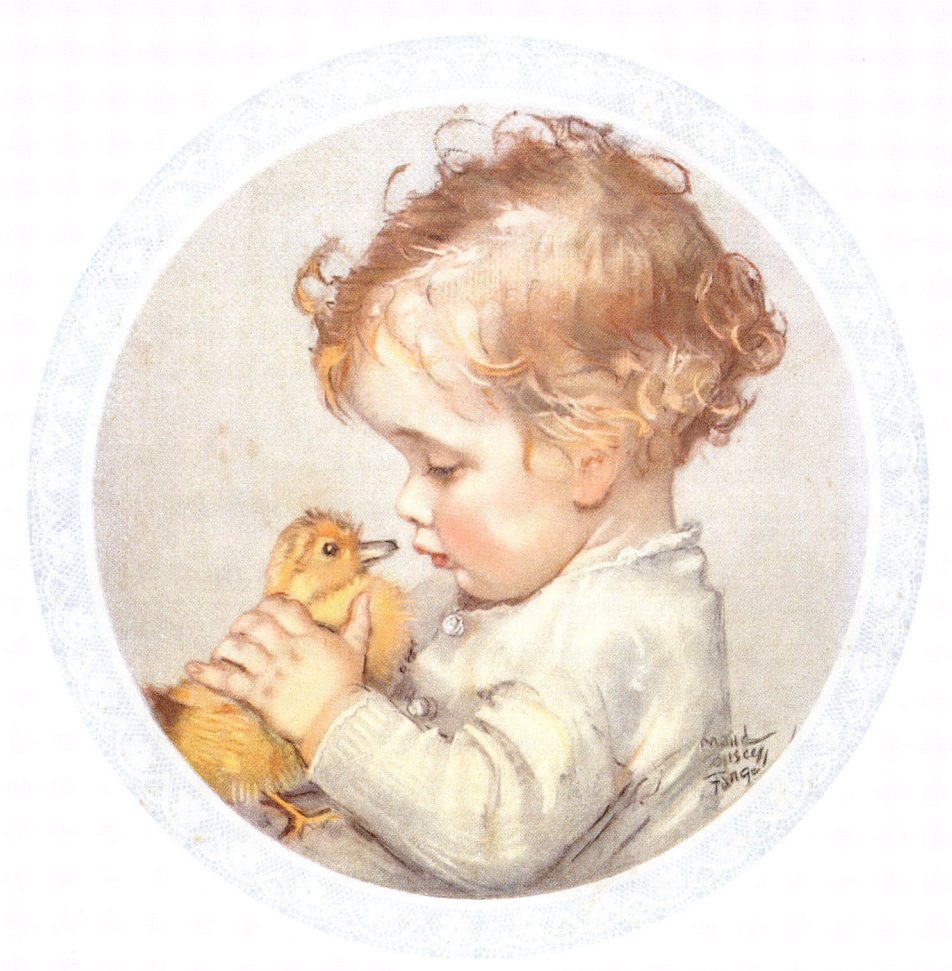

Including gentle animals.

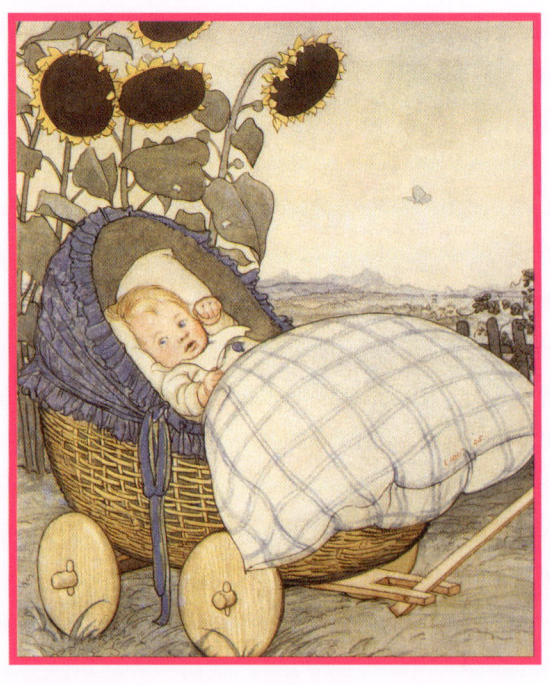

You will see and love this world in all its variety
and beauty.

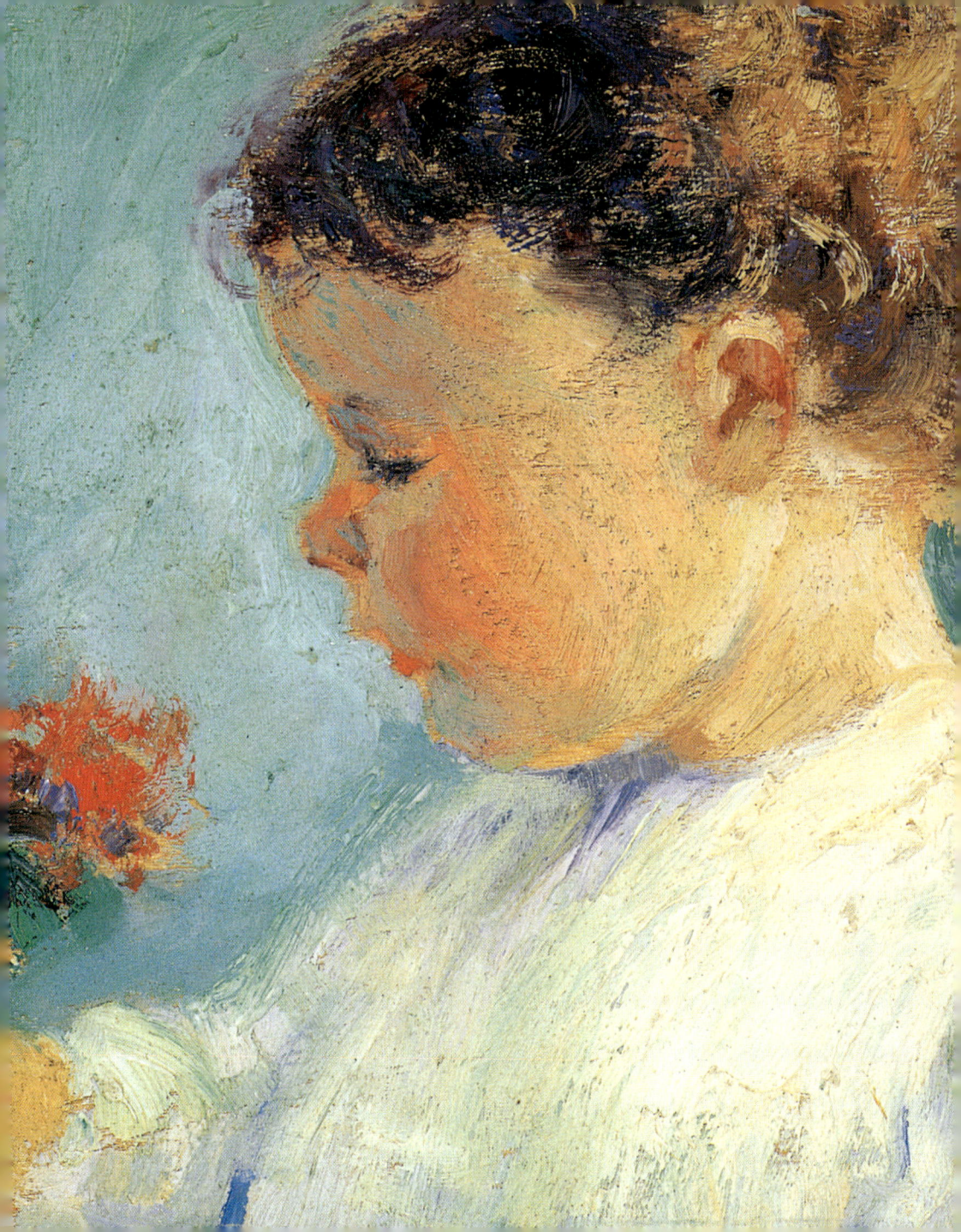

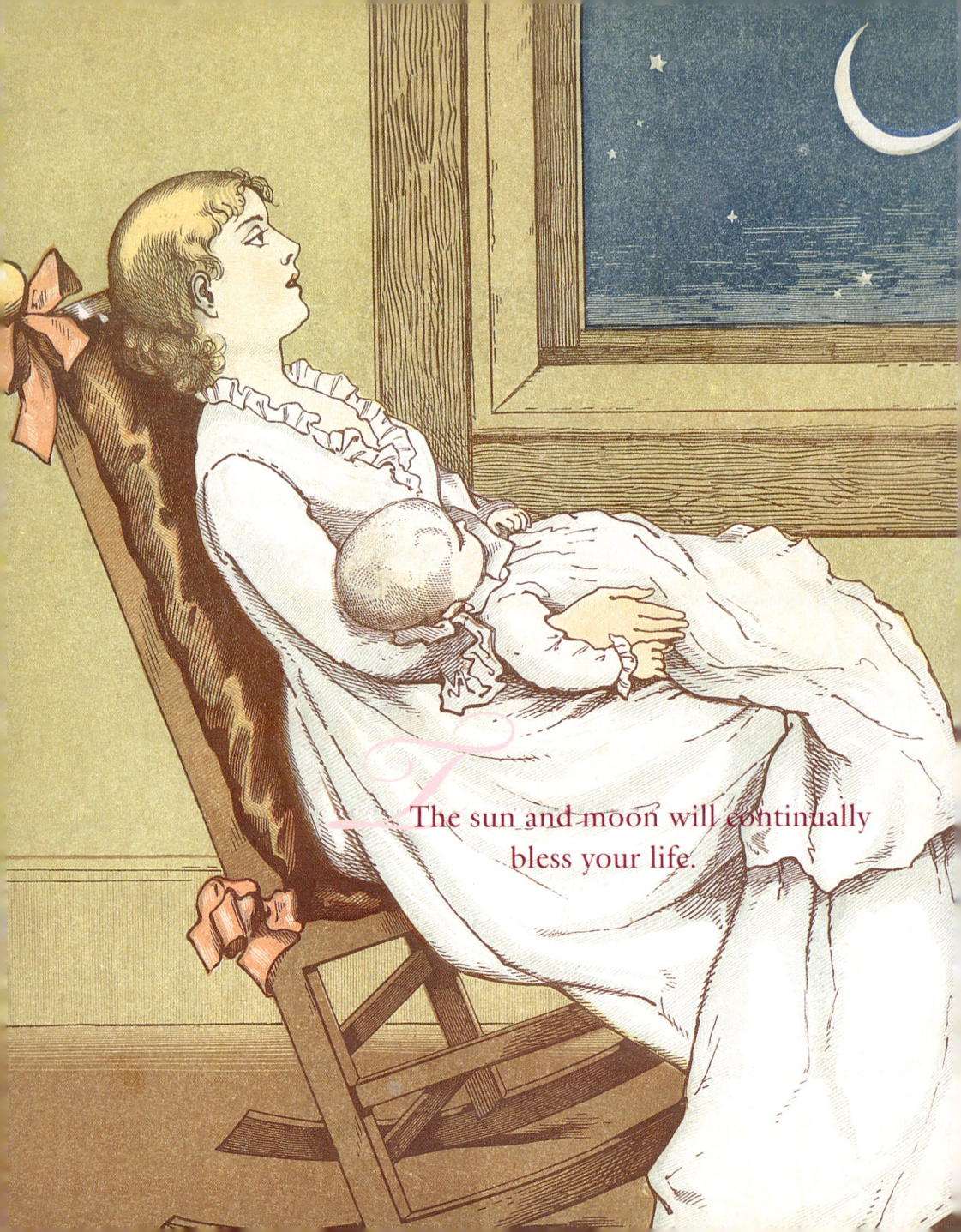

Days will hold you in their brightness,
and night enfold you in its peace.

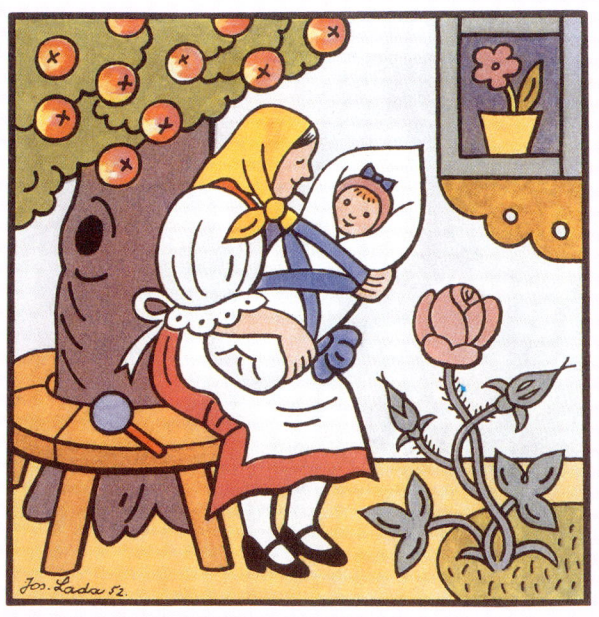

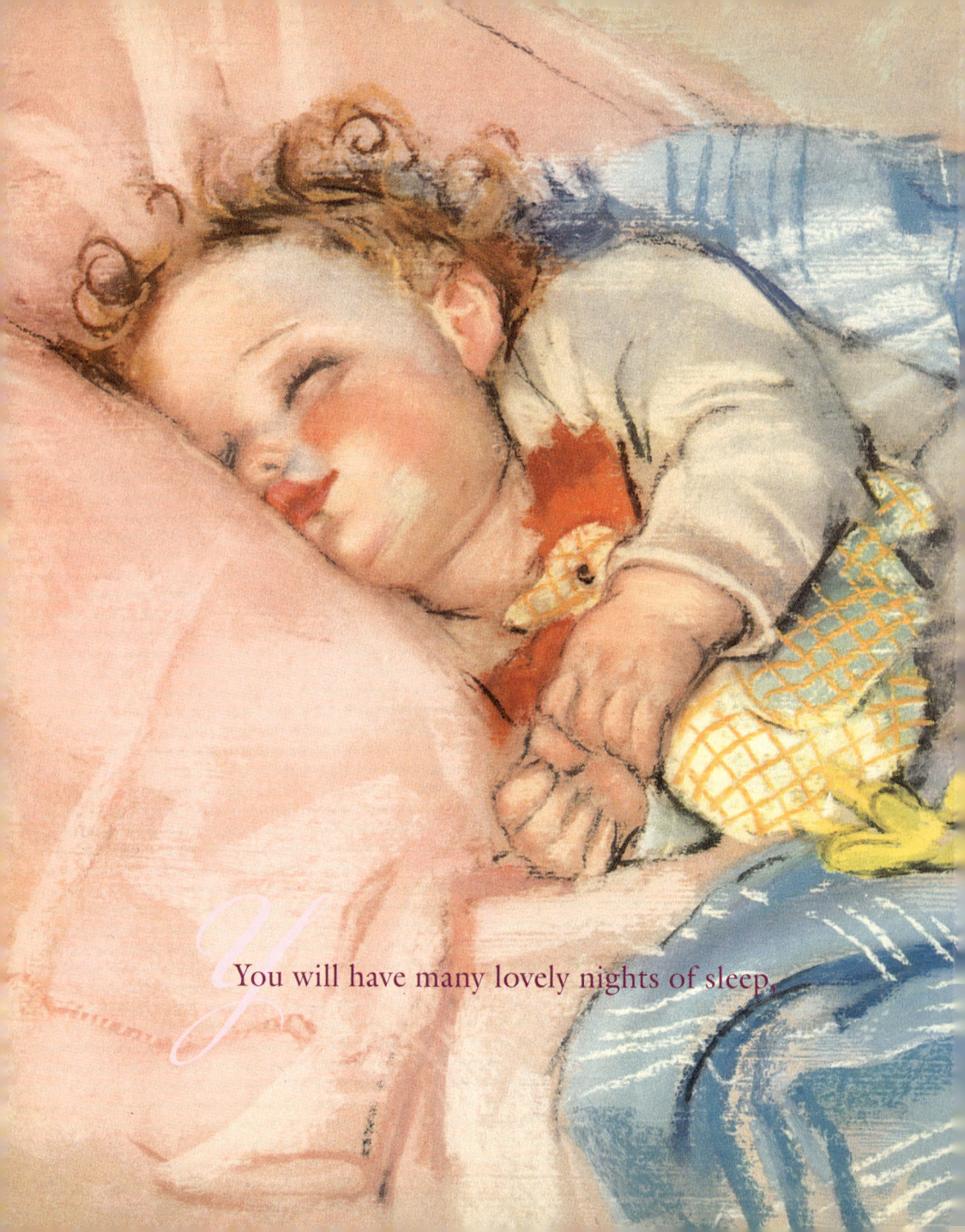

You will have many lovely nights of sleep,

And many joyful awakenings.

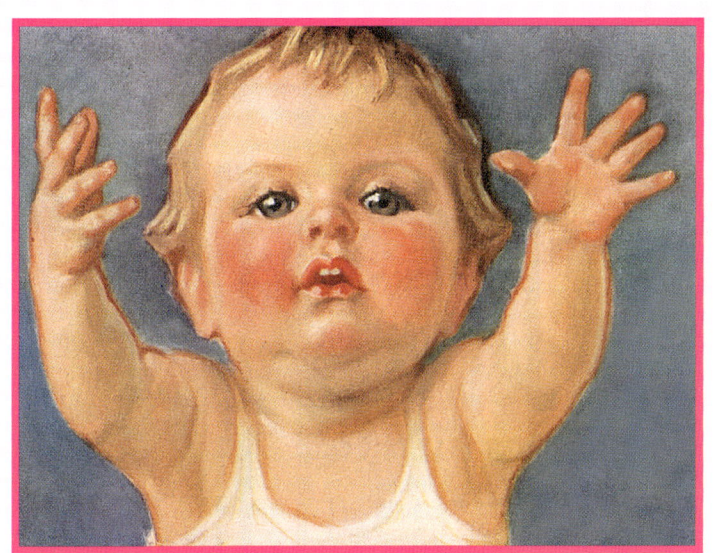

Baby – we send you all of our love, and welcome you to a glorious life.

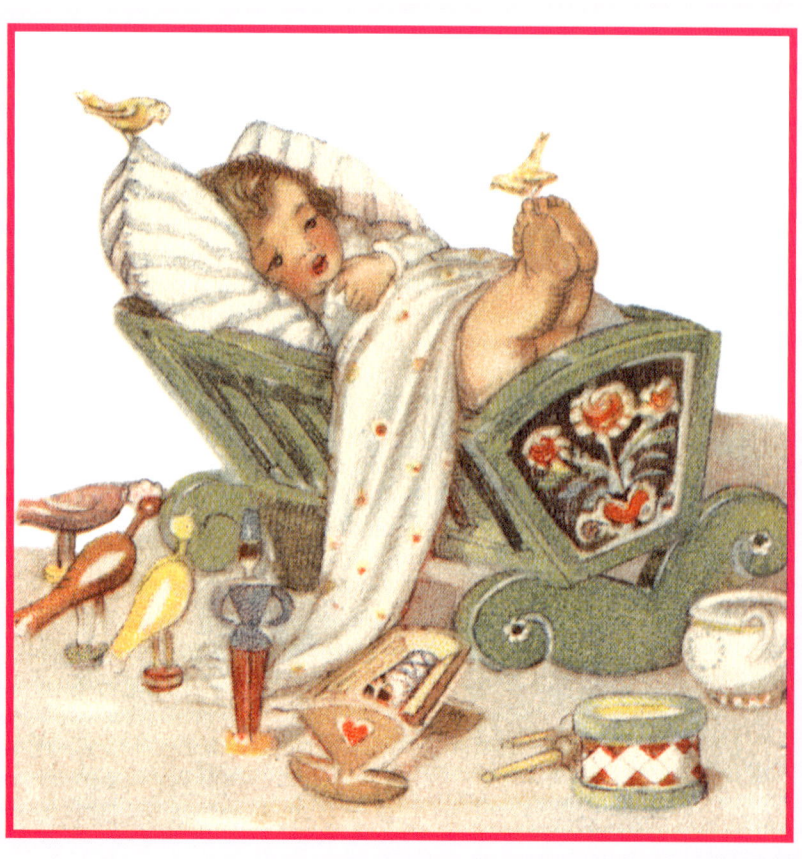

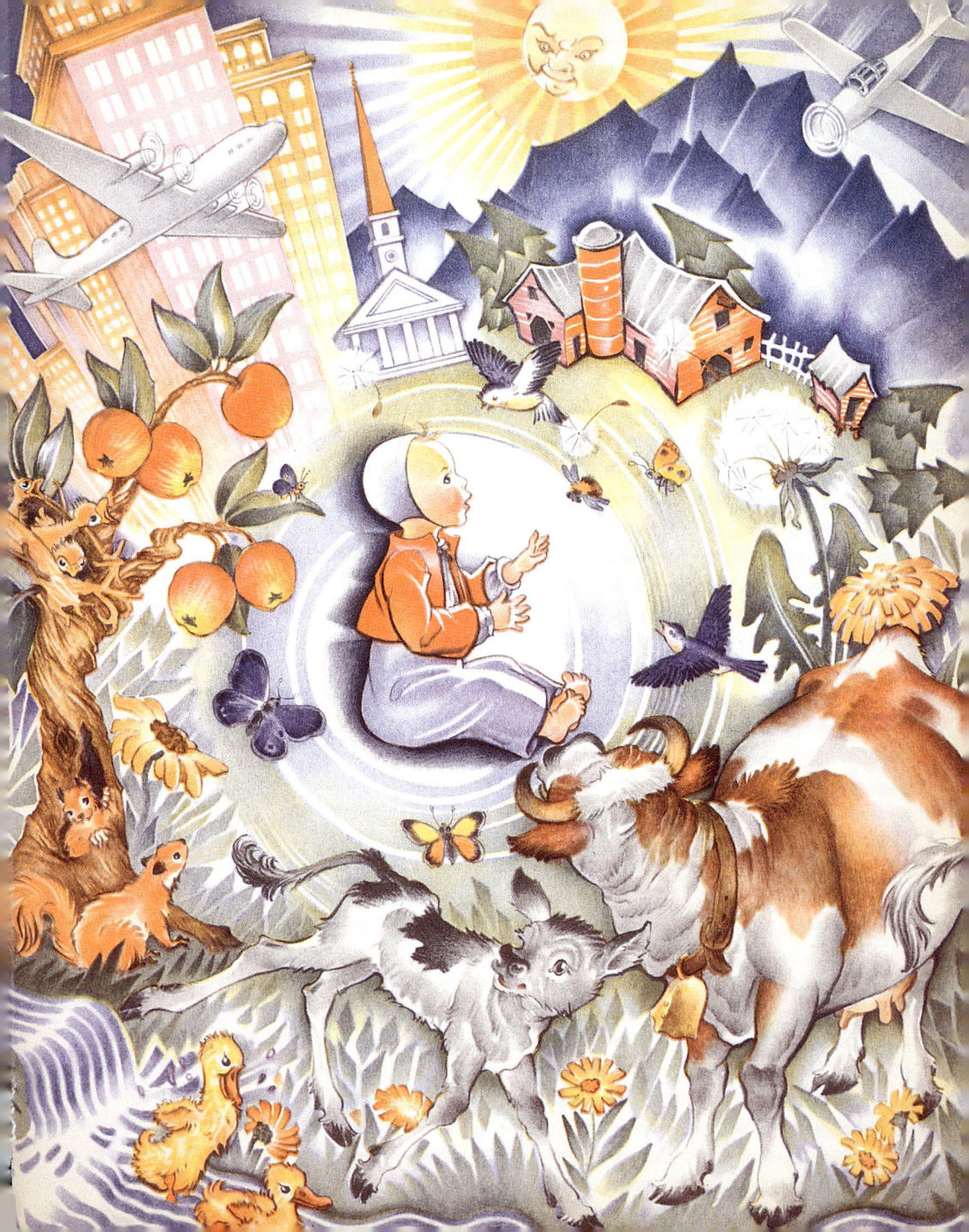

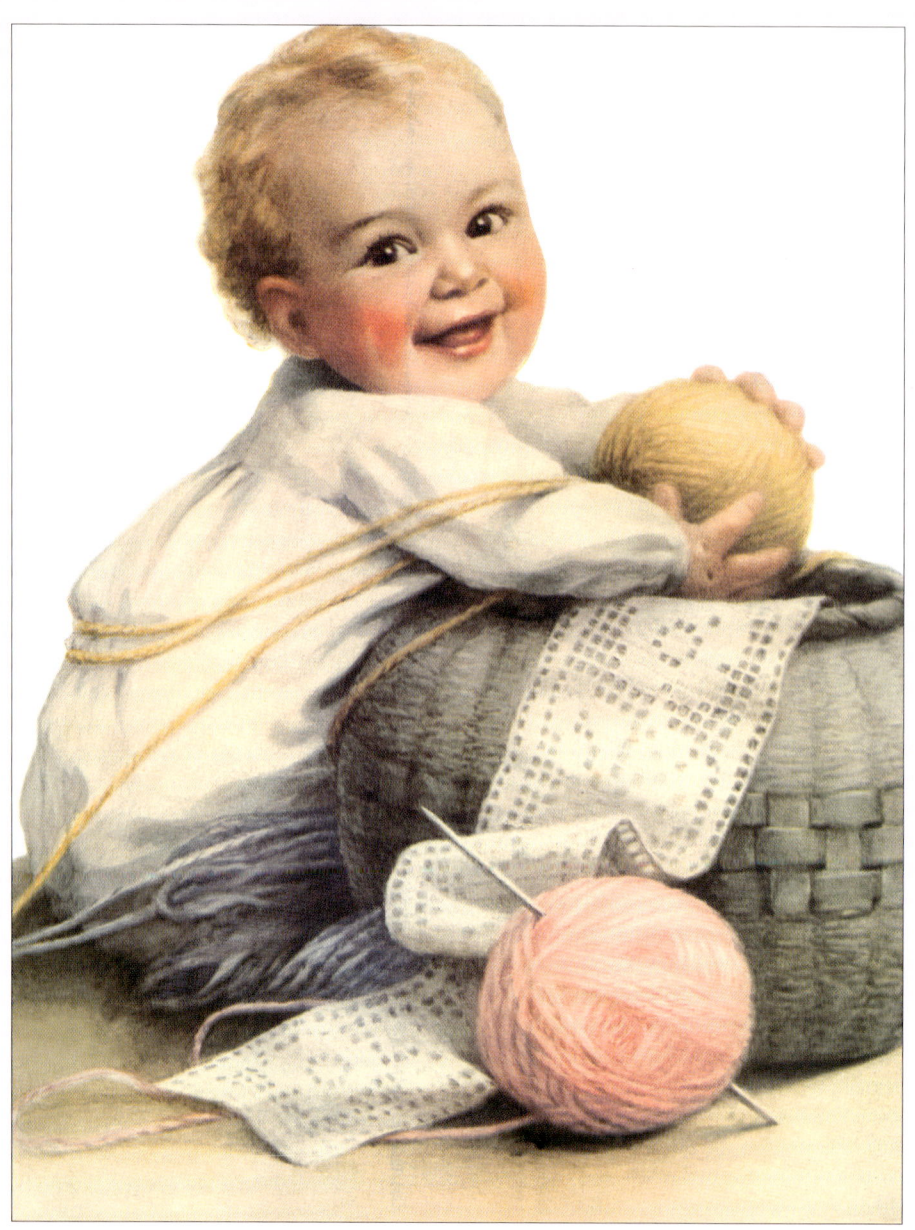

Picture Credits

Cover	Unknown. Calendar illustration, n.d.
Endpapers	Gertrud and Walther Caspari. from *Kinderhumor für Auge und Ohr*, 1908
Frontispiece	Maud and Miska Petersham. from *My Very First Book*, 1948
Title page	Unknown. Greeting card, n.d.
1	device?
2	Janice Holland. from *Bill and Susan*, 1945
3	John Gannam. Advertisement, n.d.
4	Heinrich Nauen. "Mein Garten," 1906
5	Unknown, n.d.
6	Unknown. Greeting card, n.d.
7	Ethel P.B. Leach. "Mother and Child," 1915
8	Maud Tousey Fangel. from *Babies*, 1941
9	Maud and Miska Petersham. from *My Very First Book*, 1948
10	F. Sands Brunner. Calendar illustration, 1949
11	Katherine R. Wireman. Magazine cover, 1922
12	Florence Kroger. Calendar illustration, n.d.
13	Maud Tousey Fangel. from *Babies*, 1941
14	Else Wenz-Viëtor. from *Sonnenkinder Stuben*, 1925
15	Bernhard Gutmann. "Baby," n.d.
16	Ida Waugh. from *Holly Berries*, 1881
17	Josef Lada. from *Detem*, 1960
18	Maud Tousey Fangel. Illustration, n.d.
19	Unknown. Advertisement, 1935
20	M. Fischerová-Kvechová. Postcard, n.d.
21	Maud and Miska Petersham. from *My Very First Book*, 1948
22	Annie Benson Müller. Magazine cover, 1922
Back cover	M. Hartwell. Magazine cover, 1918

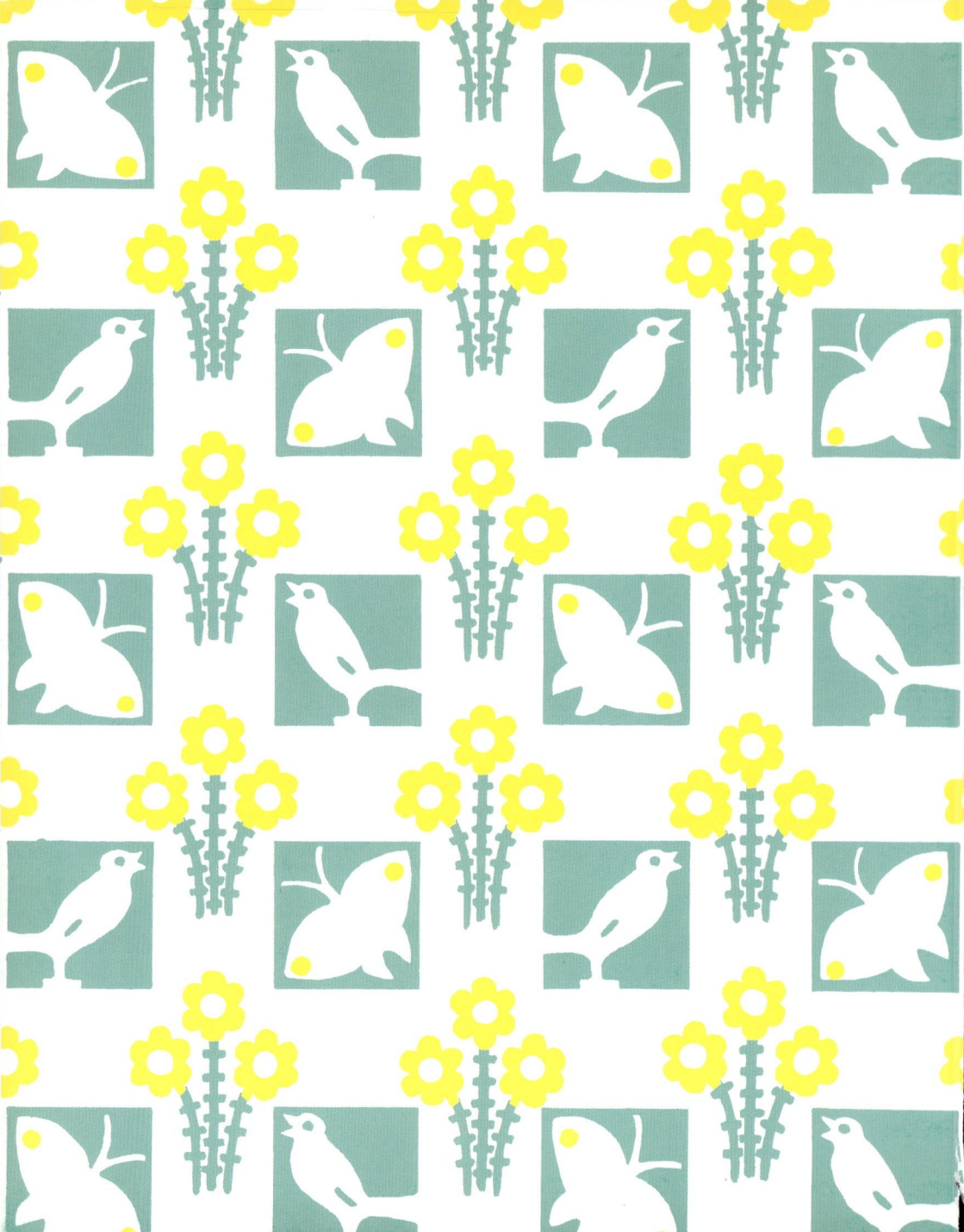